My Beautiful Teeth Series

Part 2

Let's take care of Our teeth

Dr. Tasneem Mahmoud Omran

- My Beautiful Teeth Series
- Part 2: Let's Take Care of Our Teeth
- Dr. Tasneem Mahmoud Omran
- First Edition
- All rights are reserved to the author

About this Series: Discovering the World of Dental Health

My Beautiful Teeth Series is a comprehensive and engaging guide to dental health for children aged 5-7. This 3-part series is designed to educate and inspire children to take care of their teeth, while also raising awareness about the importance of oral hygiene.

<u>1- Tiny but Mighty</u>: Explores the importance of teeth and how they help us talk and eat properly. It also teaches children about the different types of teeth and why babies don't have any teeth when they are born.

<u>2- Let's Take Care of Our Teeth</u>: Focuses on the proper techniques for brushing and flossing, as well as the importance of eating healthy foods for strong teeth.

3- A Visit to the Dentist: Takes children on a journey to the dental clinic, where they learn about the different tools and equipment used by dentists and the importance of regular check-ups.

Each book in the series contains interactive games and activities, including connect-the-dots and matching exercises that will keep children engaged and entertained while learning about dental health. Additionally, a QR code included in each book, allows children to play each game in an interactive way using their mobile phone or tablet.

"My Beautiful Teeth Series" is a must-have for any parent looking to educate their children about dental health in a fun and engaging way.

Clean Teeth, Clean Mouth, Clean Body

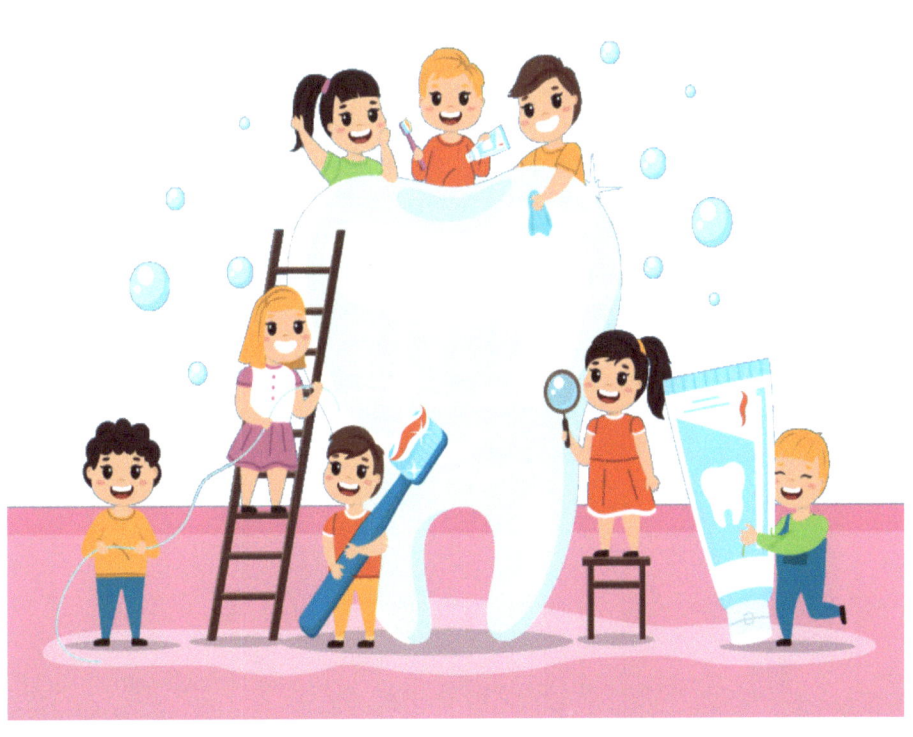

How do we keep ourselves clean?

We wash our hands before we eat and after using the bathroom.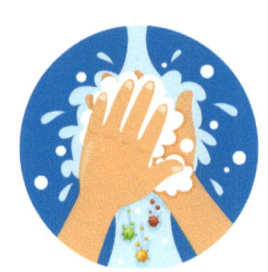

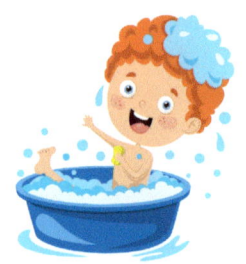 We take a bath or shower to get clean all over.

We wear clean clothes every day.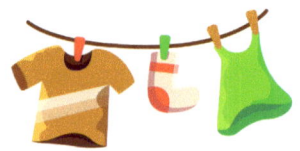

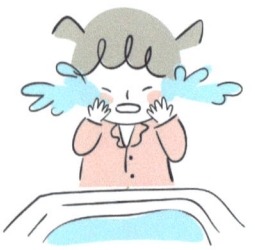 We wash our face every morning and night.

When we keep ourselves clean, we stay healthy and smell good.

It's important to clean our bodies and clothes regularly so we don't get sick.

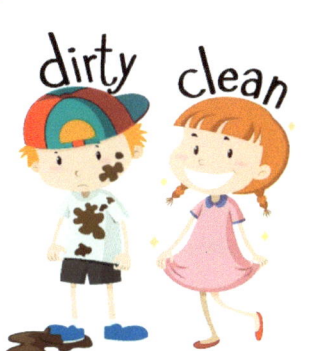

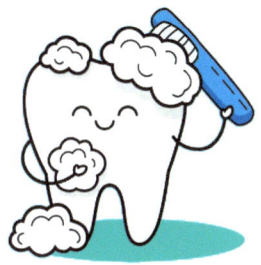

Our teeth are also part of our body. So, it's important to keep them clean too!

We should also scrub our tongues because dirty tongue can smell bad.

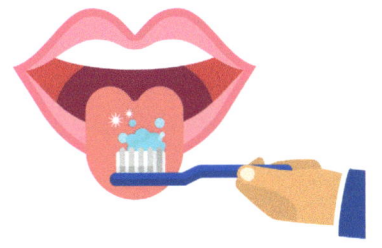

We clean our teeth using a toothbrush that is the right size for our mouths. We should brush our teeth twice a day.

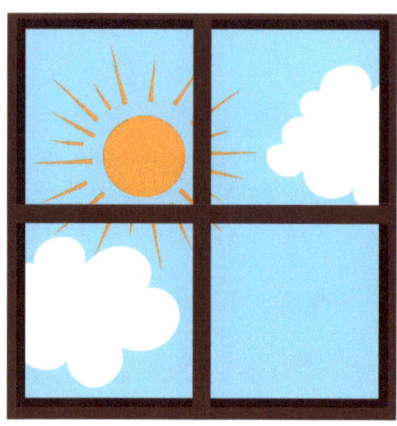 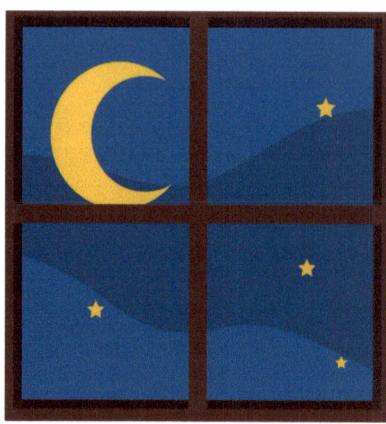

In the morning   At night, before going to bed

We put a small amount of toothpaste on our toothbrush.

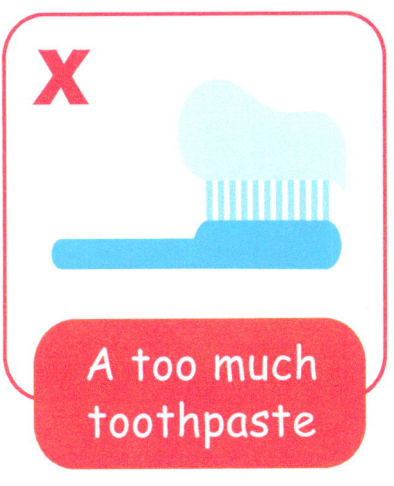

A too much toothpaste

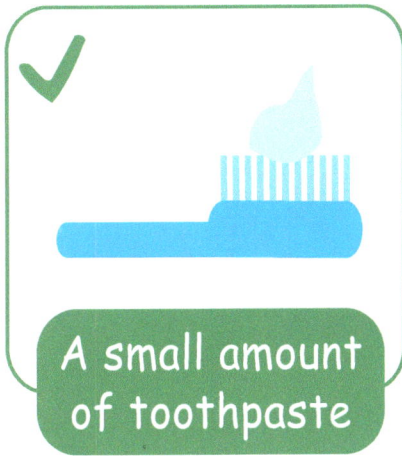

A small amount of toothpaste

Toothpaste has a special ingredient called Fluoride that helps make our teeth stronger.

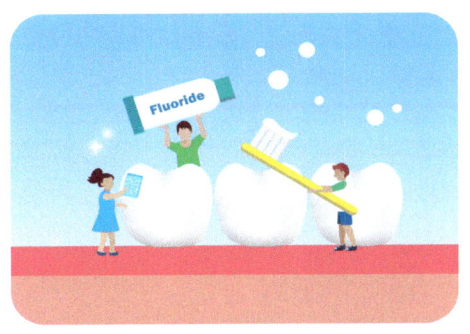

Toothpaste works better than just water to clean our teeth and make our mouths taste good.

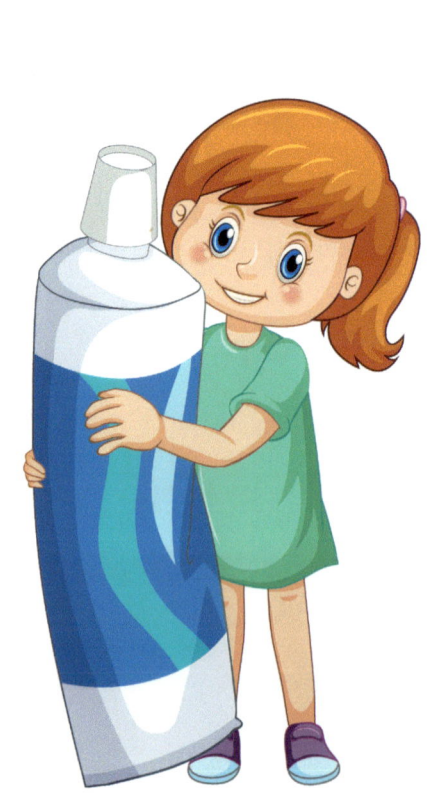

For little kids (younger than 3 years): We use a tiny amount, like a grain of rice.

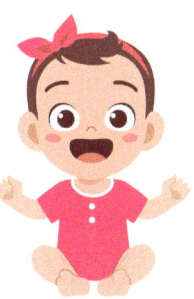

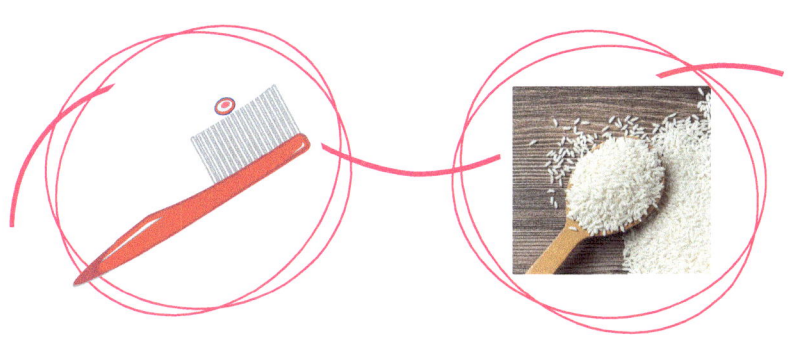

For older kids (older than 3 years): We use a small amount, like a green pea.

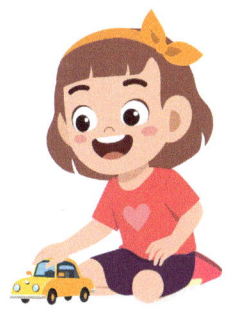

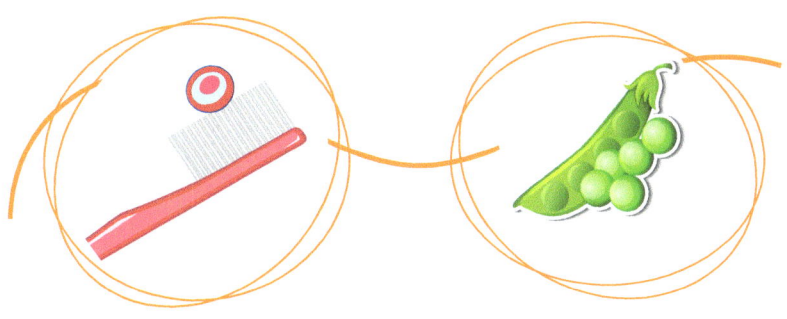

When we brush our teeth, we should not swallow the toothpaste. We should spit it out.

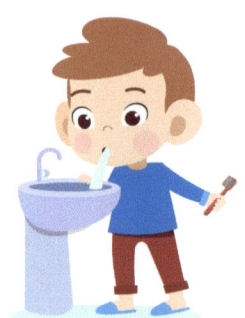

Toothpaste is for cleaning our teeth, not our stomachs.

We need to brush the inside, outside, and top of each tooth.

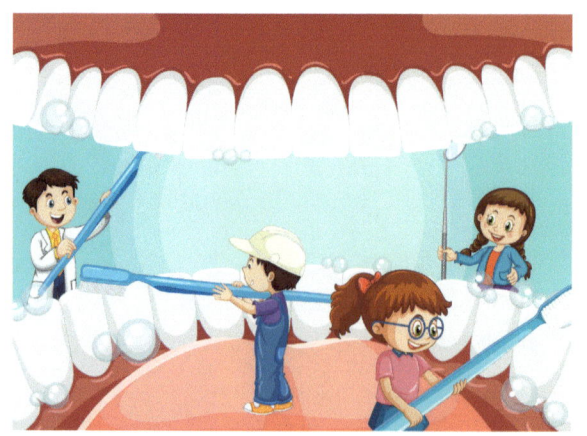

The outside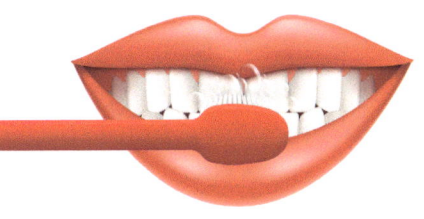

The inside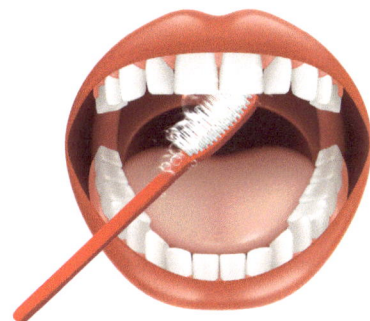

The top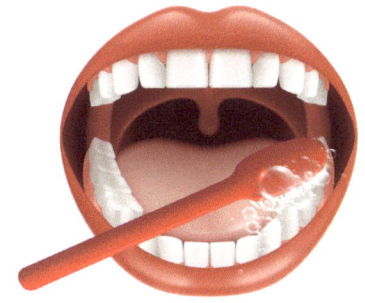

We should move the toothbrush back and forth gently.

Your mom, dad, or another grown-up may help you brush your teeth.

Brushing our teeth is not enough to keep them clean.

We also need to clean between our teeth, just like how we clean between our fingers.

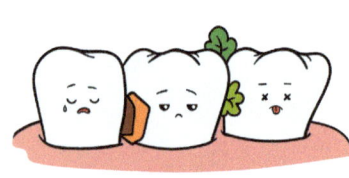 A toothbrush is too big to clean between our teeth. It's too tight there.

That's why we use floss to clean between our teeth.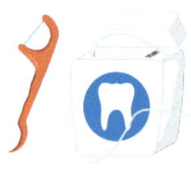

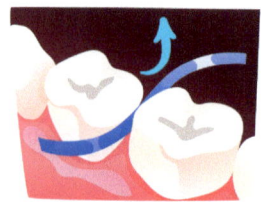 Mom, dad or another grown-up can help you floss your teeth.

Choose a toothbrush that is the right size for your mouth and easy for you to hold.

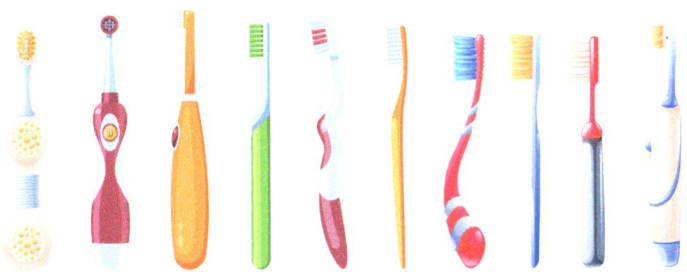

Remember to get a new toothbrush every 3 months. Old toothbrushes are not good for our teeth.

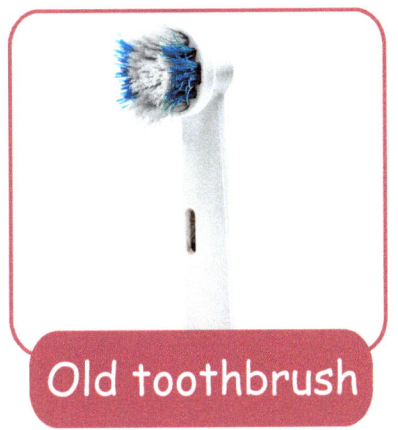
Old toothbrush

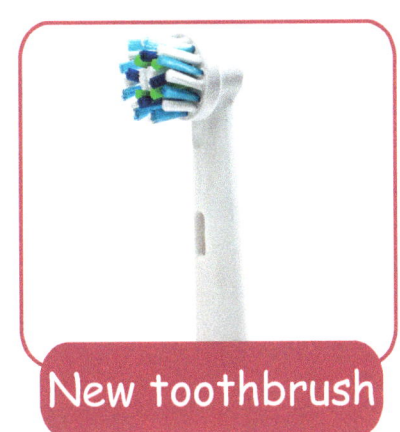
New toothbrush

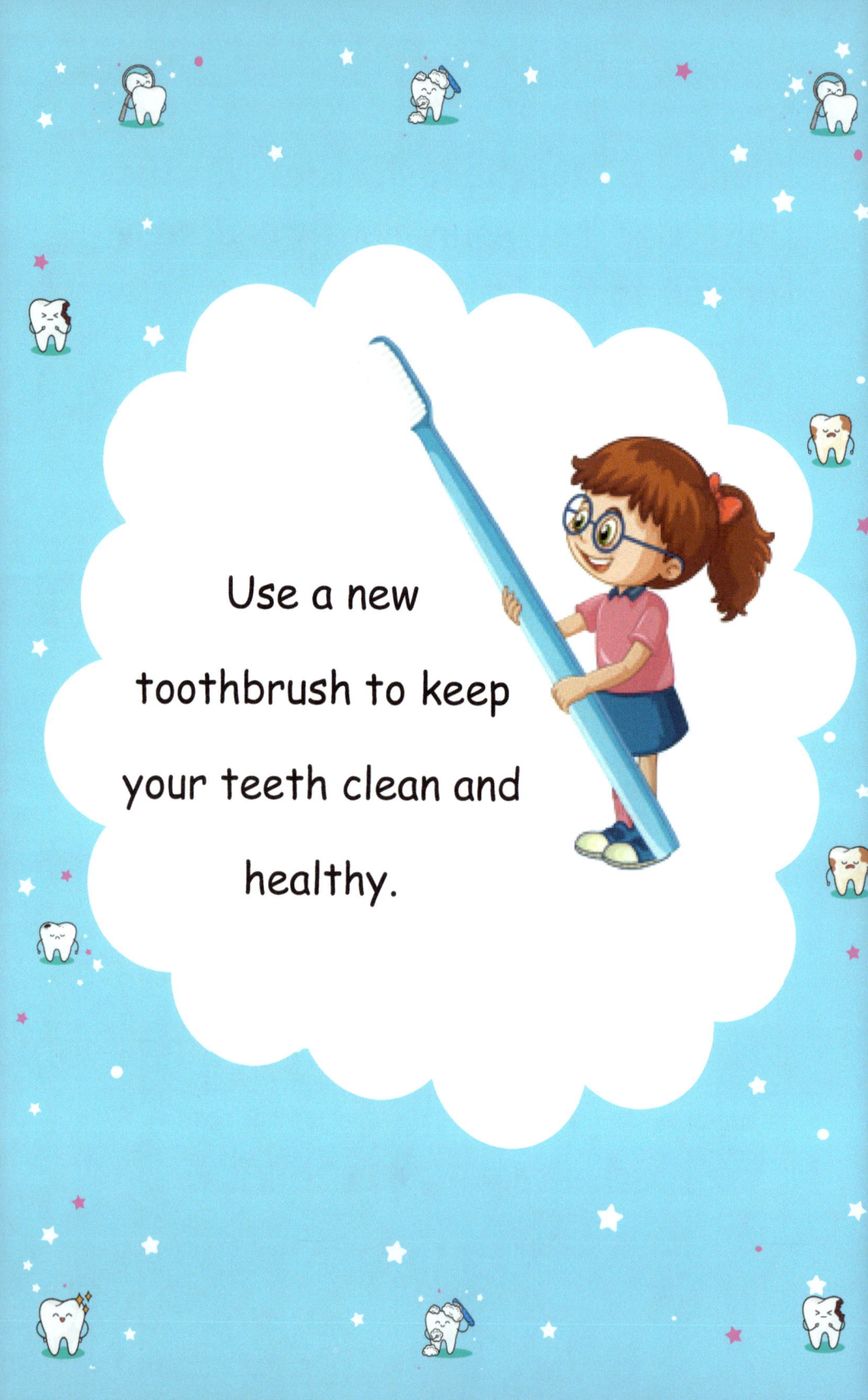

Let's Play

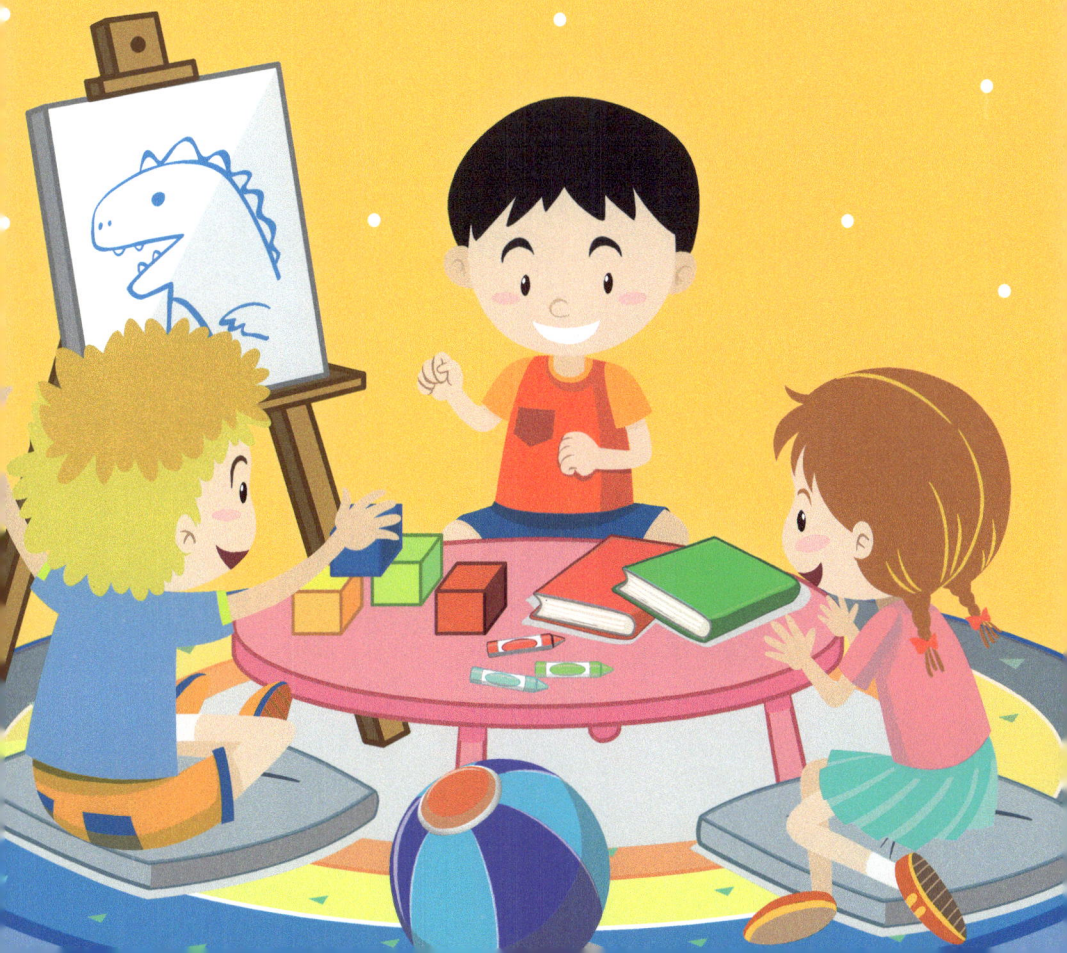

Connect the dots from 1 to 20 to reveal a fun picture!

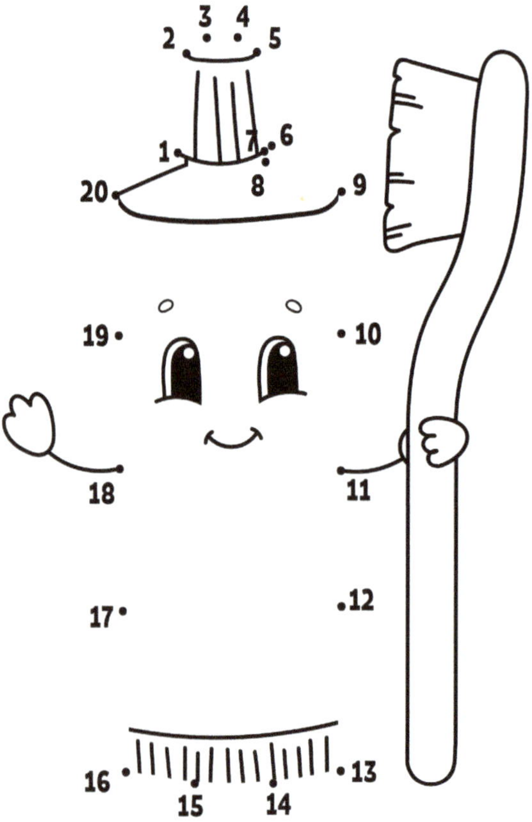

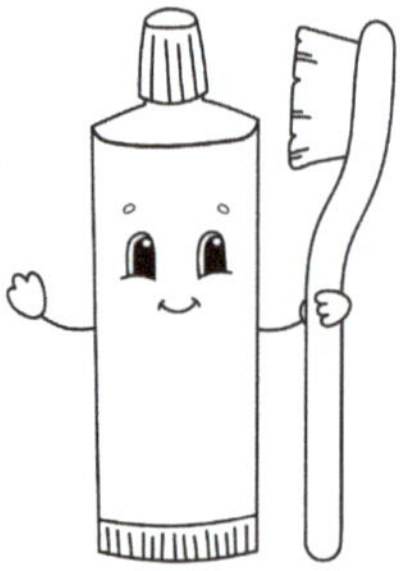

Follow the numbers in the right order to guide the tooth to the brushing station!

			38	24	78	28	80	48	98
			79	7	8	9	10	58	90
			1	6	3	27	11	12	30
31	32	1	34	5	36	37	8	13	40
41	42	2	3	4	46	47	15	14	50
88	26	53	14	13	12	17	16	59	60
61	62	63	21	20	19	18	68	69	70
74	72	73	22	17	18	77			
81	82	83	23	24	25	20			
91	64	93	94	95	26	27			

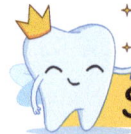 Select the right picture:

What do we use to clean our teeth?

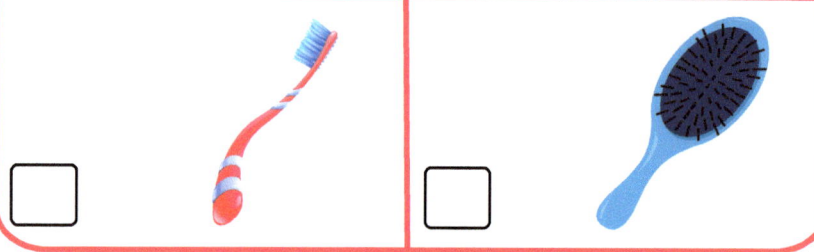

What do we put on the toothbrush?

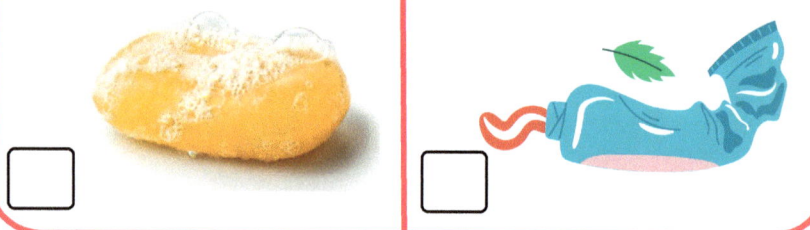

What do we use to clean between our teeth?

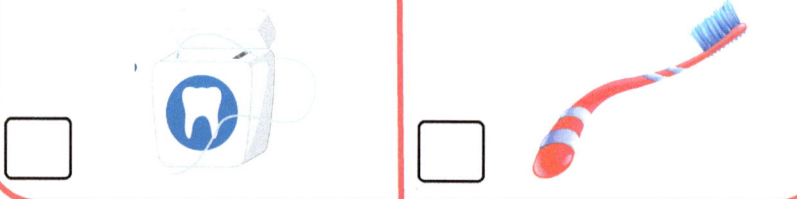

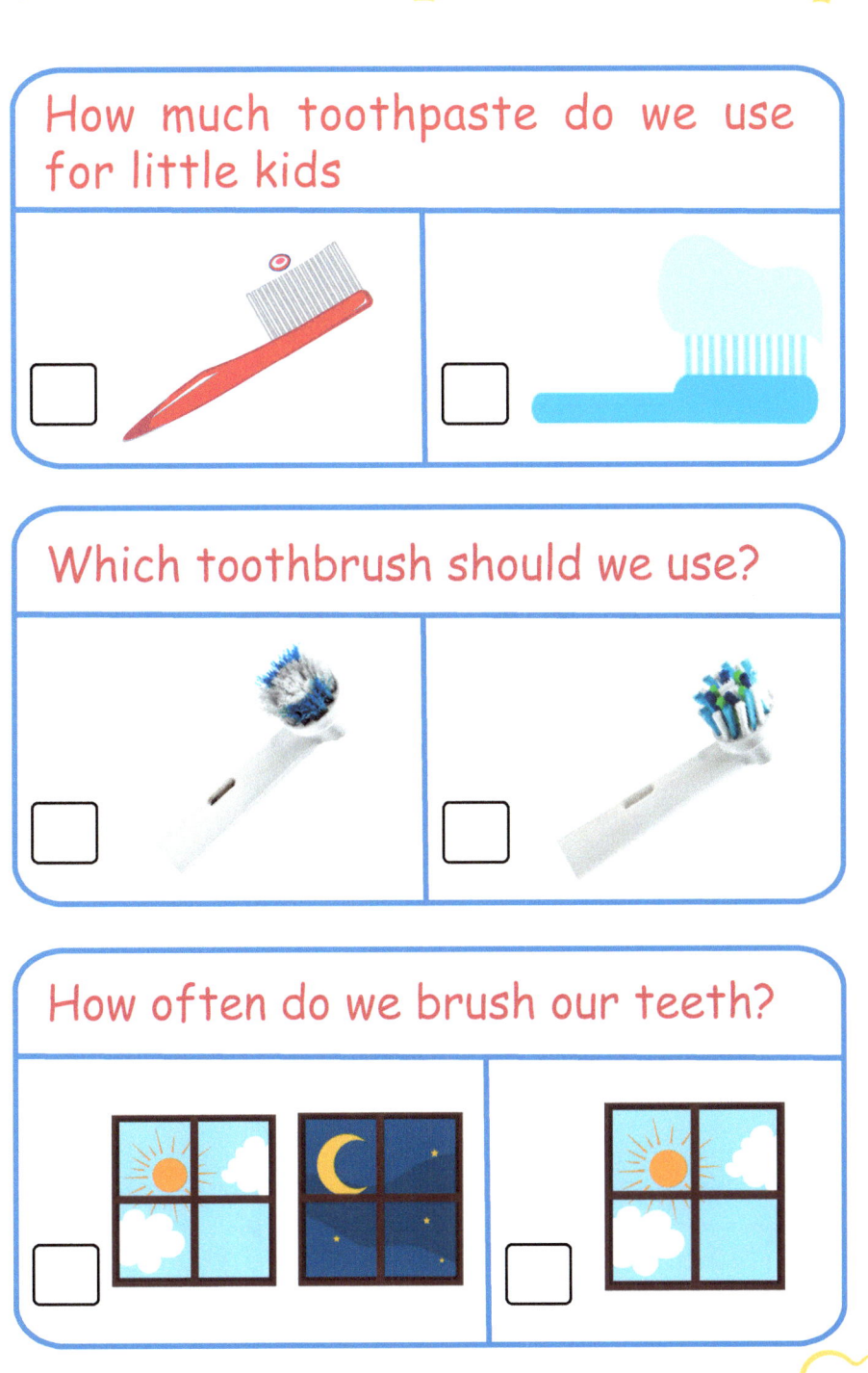

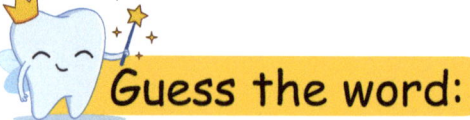 Guess the word:

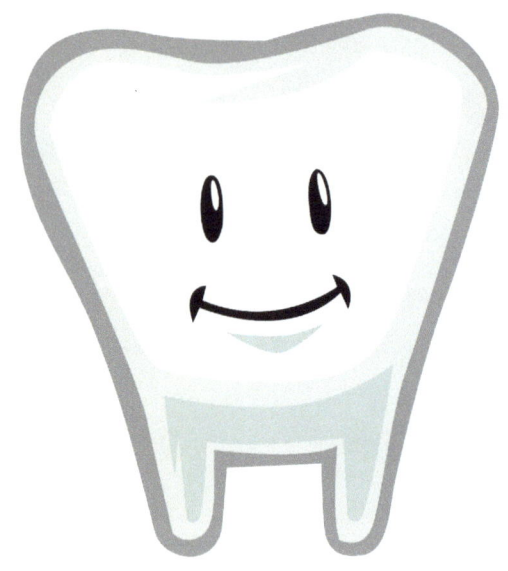

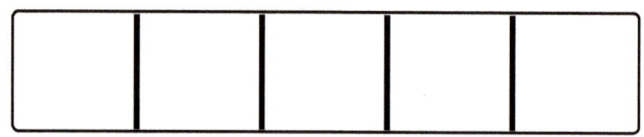

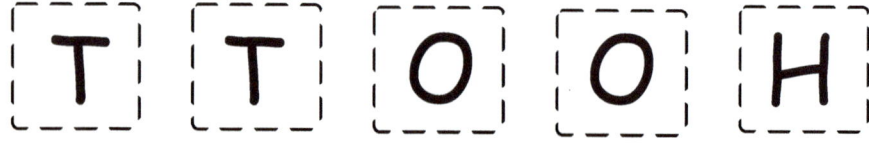

Why is it important to clean our teeth?

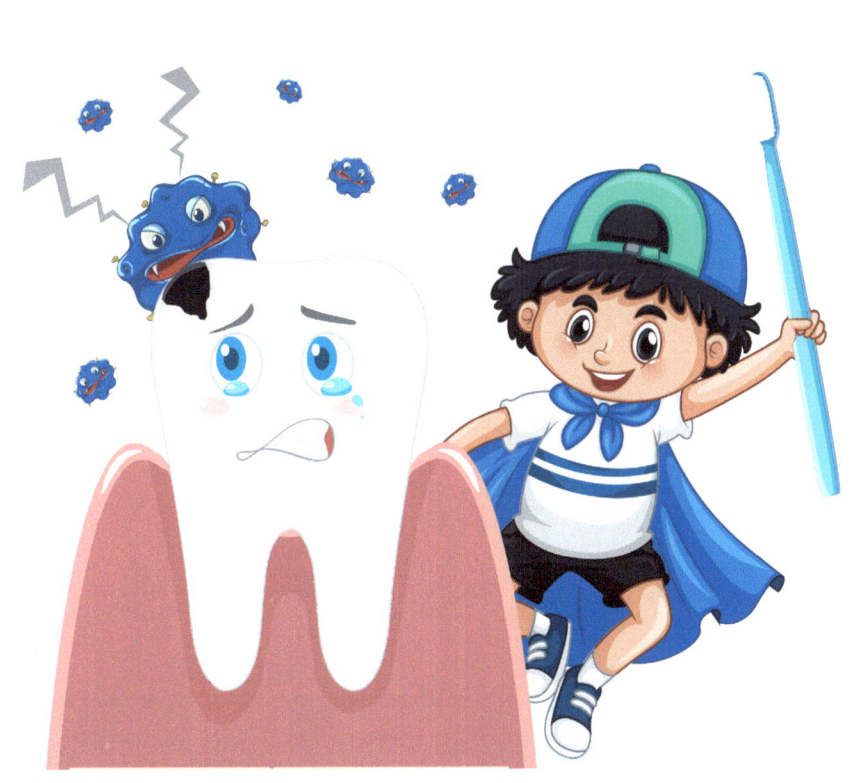

Think back to the last time you forgot to brush your teeth before going to bed.

How did your mouth feel when you woke up the next morning?

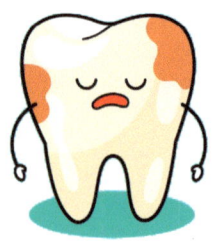

Were your teeth feeling sticky or slimy?

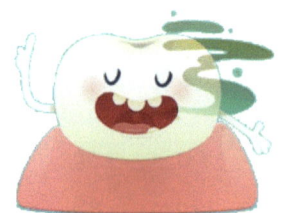

Did your breath smell bad?

That's because there's something else that sticks to our teeth besides the food we eat.

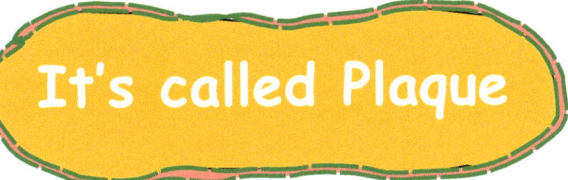

It's called Plaque

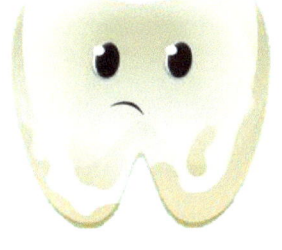

But what is plaque?

Plaque is a thin, clear film that we can't see, but it builds up on our teeth all the time.

It's full of germs that can harm our teeth.

If we don't brush the plaque off our teeth, these germs can create tiny holes in our teeth called cavities.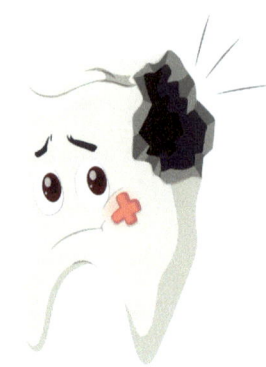

This can make our teeth hurt and weaker.

That's why it's so important to brush all the plaque off our teeth every day to keep them healthy and strong.

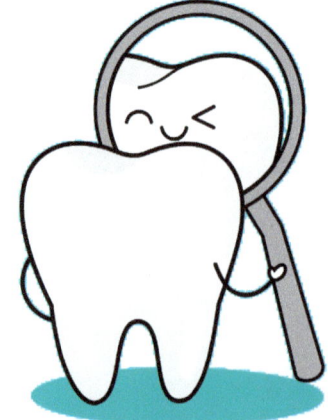

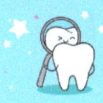

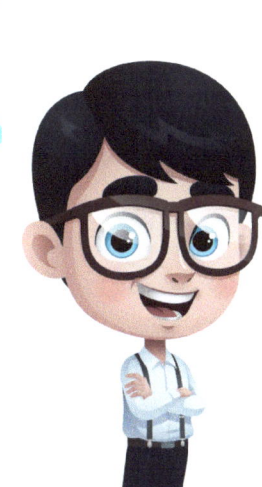

Do you remember how many times per day should you brush your teeth?

Let's Play

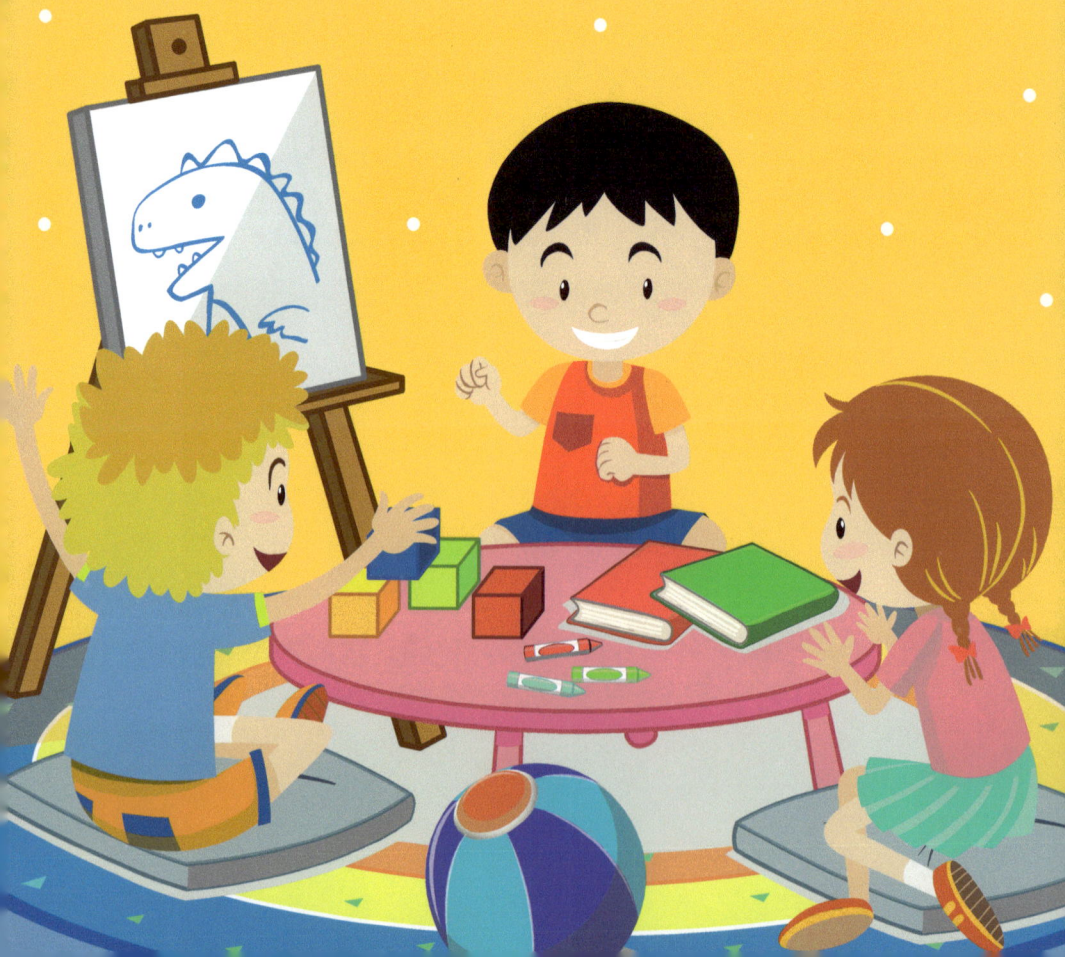

Choose the two missing pieces to complete the picture:

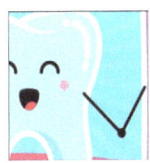 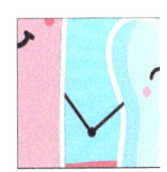 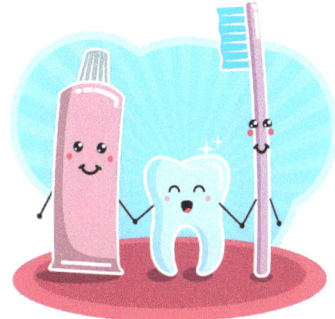

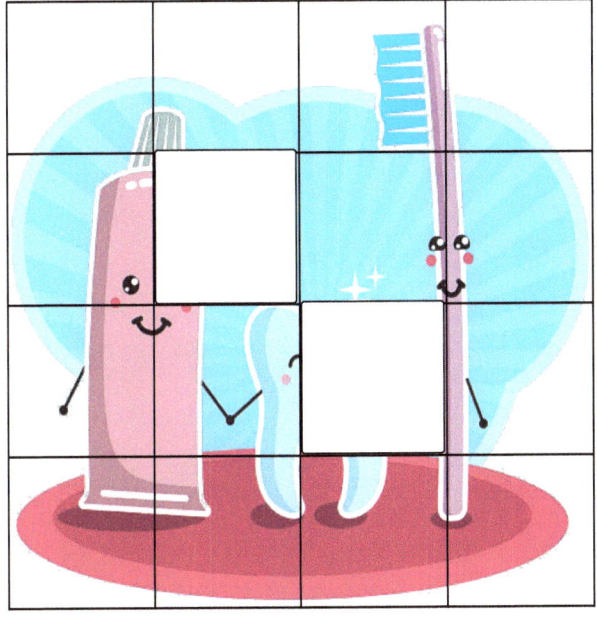 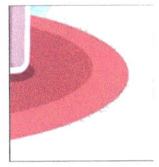

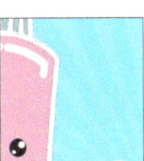

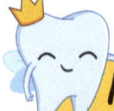 

Match the pictures with their shadows:

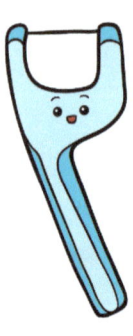 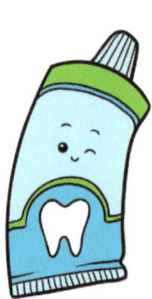 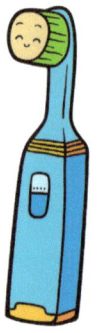 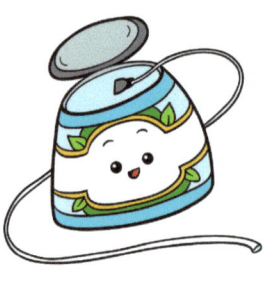

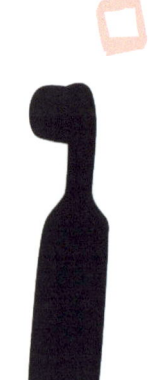 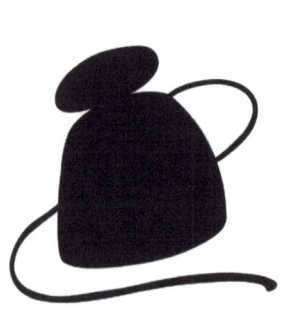 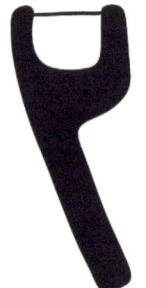 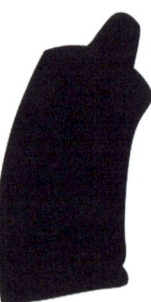

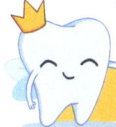

Dental Discovery: Word Search

L	T	A	M	X	U	Q	J	K	T
Q	O	A	H	I	F	D	Z	O	O
G	O	S	A	E	L	Y	O	C	O
D	T	I	B	M	O	E	R	A	T
P	H	U	J	T	S	Z	P	V	H
L	B	M	V	B	S	G	G	I	P
A	R	X	O	A	D	E	V	T	A
Q	U	D	E	Q	O	R	R	Y	S
U	S	N	Z	B	Y	M	X	L	T
E	H	A	O	C	P	S	G	Y	E

Find the following words in the puzzle:

- TOOTHPASTE
- PLAQUE
- GERMS
- TOOTHBRUSH
- CAVITY
- FLOSS

Healthy Food, Healthy Teeth

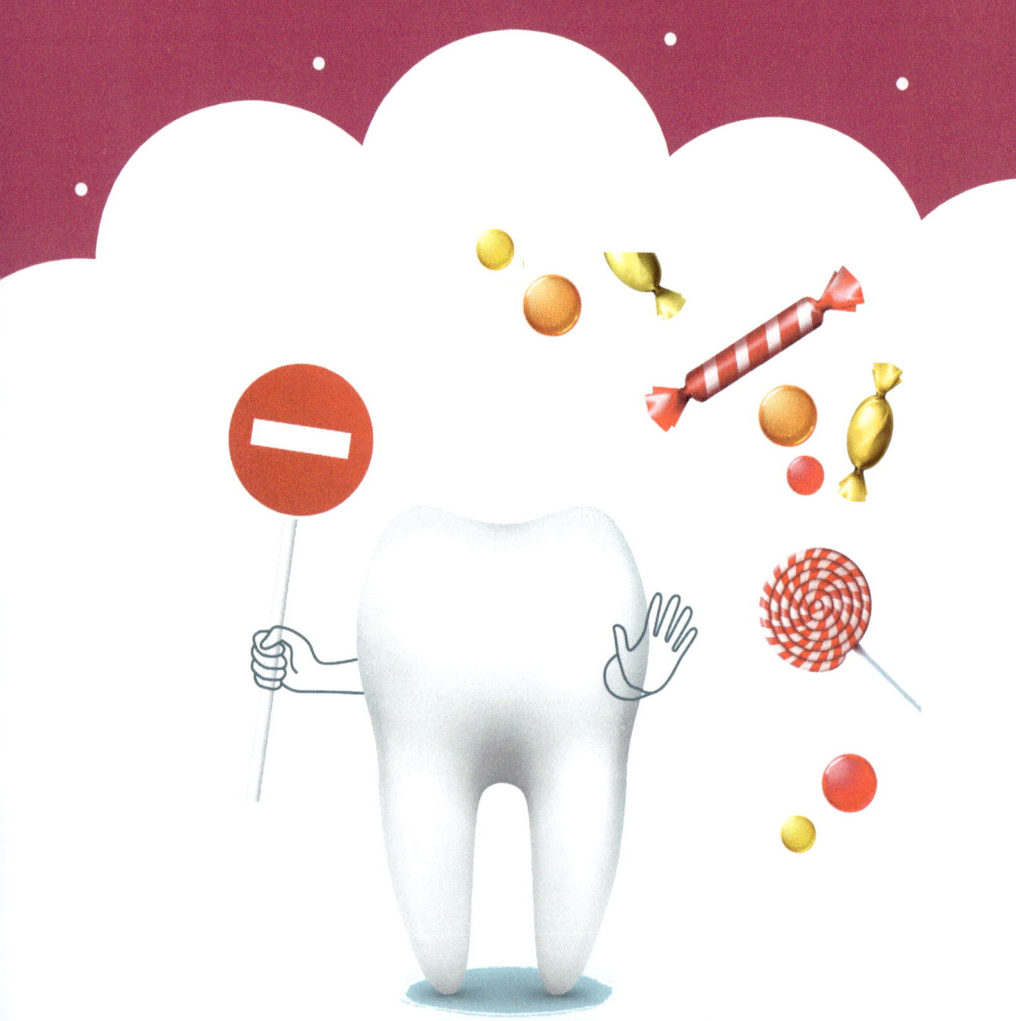

Do you want to keep your teeth strong and healthy?

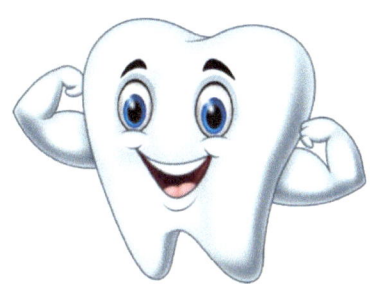

It's not just about brushing and flossing, it's also about what you eat and drink.

The foods we eat are just as important for keeping our teeth healthy as they are for keeping our bodies healthy.

Eating a mix of healthy foods for breakfast, lunch, and dinner is the best way to keep your teeth and whole body in good shape.

When you're hungry and need a snack, choose foods like fruit, cheese, yogurt, or raw vegetables.

Drink water or milk when you're thirsty. Try to avoid sugary drinks and sweets.

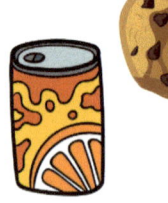

If you do have sweets, it's best to eat them with your meals.

Examples of healthy food:

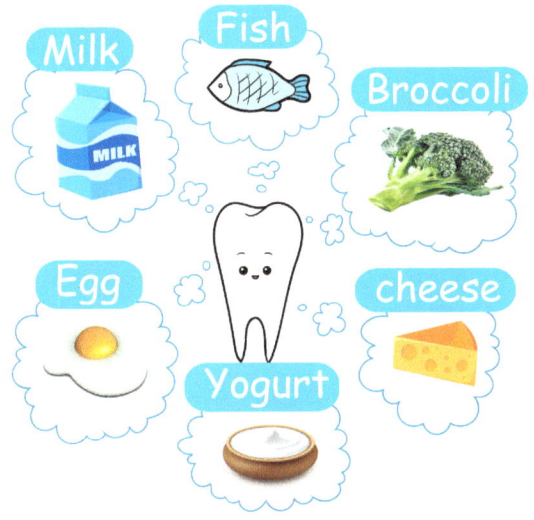

Examples of unhealthy food:

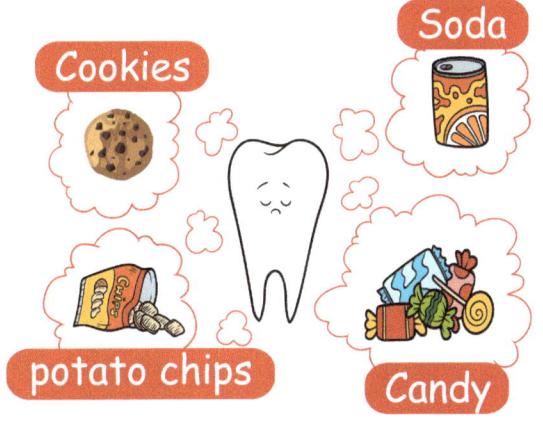

Now we know how important it is to keep our teeth clean.

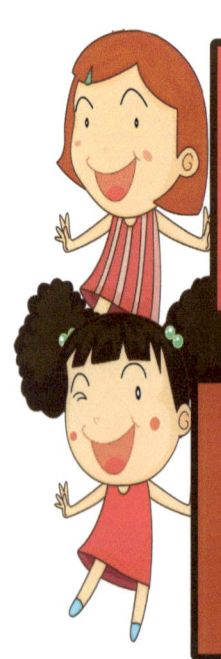

We should brush two times a day and floss once a day to remove plaque.

And we should also eat healthy foods to keep our teeth strong and healthy.

Let's Play

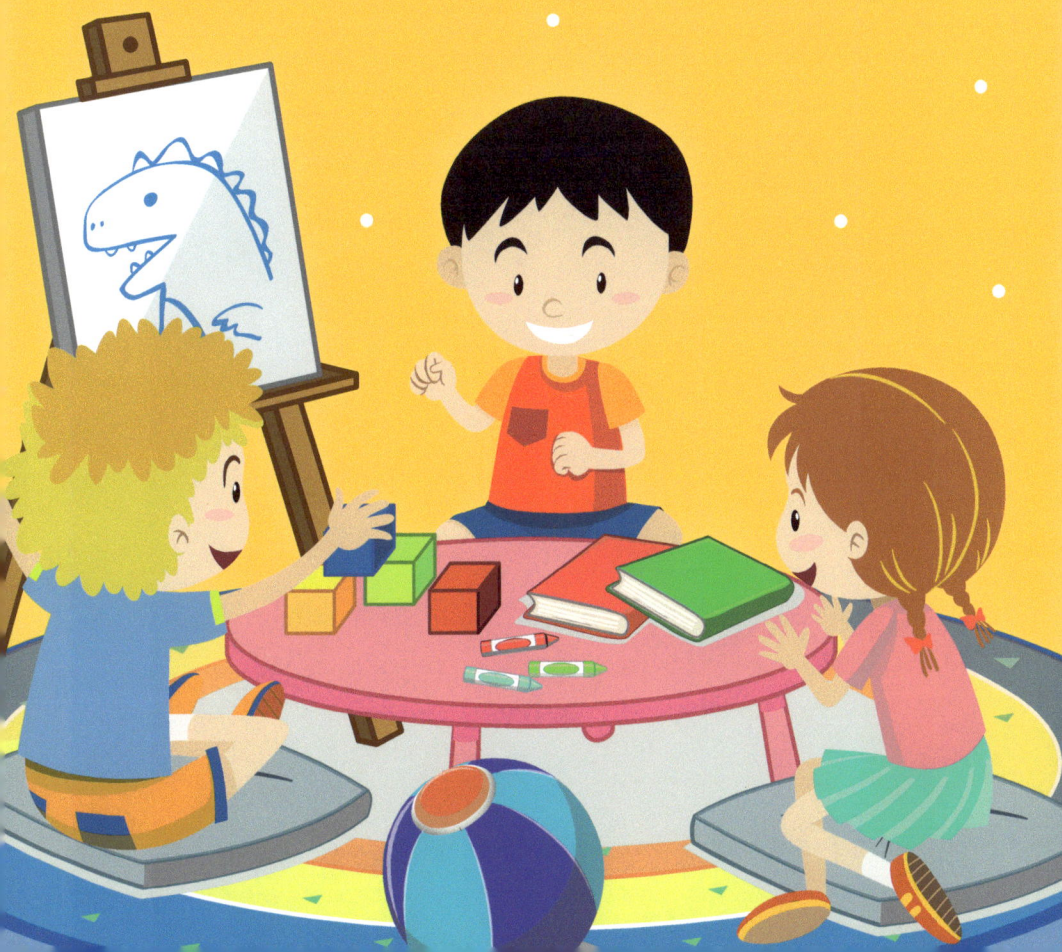

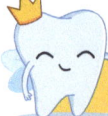 Place the food items in the correct column: healthy or unhealthy

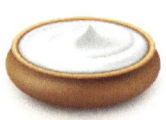  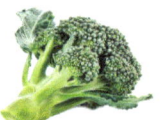 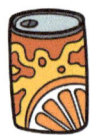

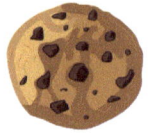 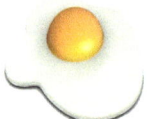 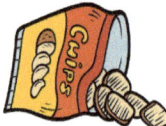 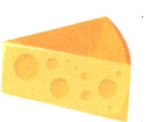

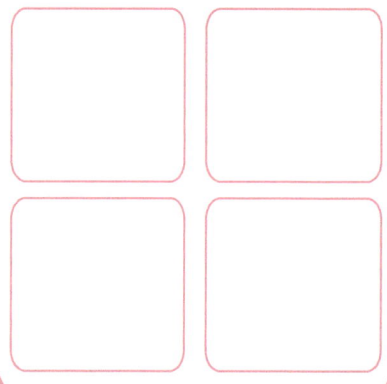

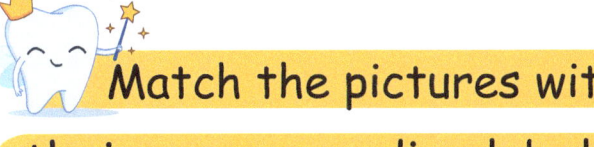 **Match the pictures with their corresponding labels**

Tongue Brushing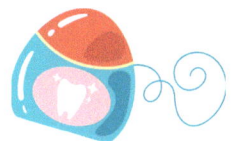

Eating Healthy Food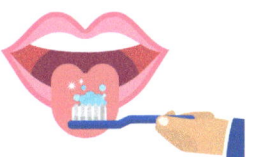

Flossing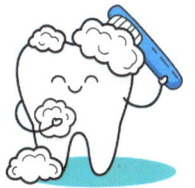

Teeth Brushing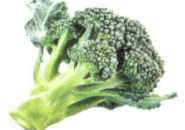

Color the correct number of items in each row

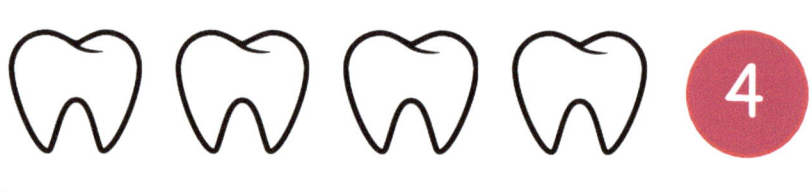
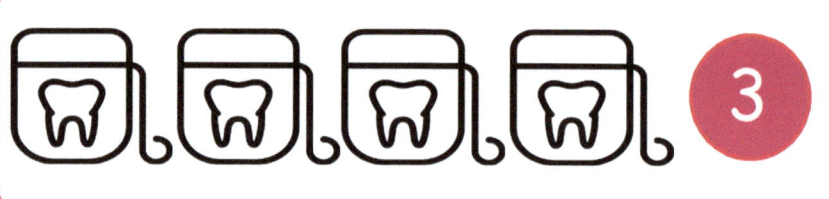
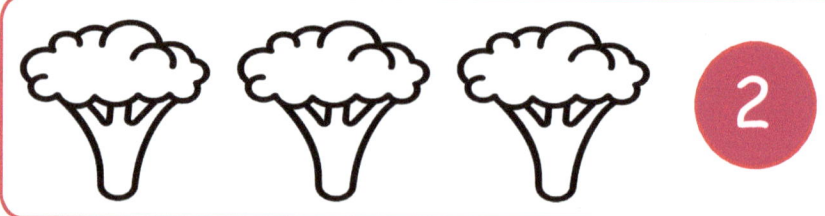

Guide to the parents

About the book:

This book is designed to help your child understand the importance of oral hygiene and the steps they can take to maintain healthy teeth and gums. By the end of the book, your child will have a better understanding of:

- The reasons why we should clean our teeth.
- The proper techniques for cleaning our teeth.
- The types of food that are best for our teeth.

To get the most out of this interactive book, we recommend the following:

• Preview the book before reading it with your child to familiarize yourself with the content.

• Bring energy and enthusiasm to your reading sessions with your child.

• Take breaks to ask your child questions and discuss what you've read together.

• Use the games and activities provided at the end of each section to assess your child's comprehension.

- Consider revisiting the book with your child for added reinforcement.

- Take advantage of the QR codes provided throughout the book. These codes can be scanned with a smart device for an interactive and fun learning experience.

Some helpful dental information:

1. Parents should start their child's dental hygiene from birth by massaging the gums twice a day. When the first tooth appears, parents should begin brushing their child's teeth twice a day and avoid letting the child fall asleep with a bottle in the mouth.

2. The recommended fluoride concentration in children's toothpaste is 1000 PPM.

3. For children under 3 years old, use a grain of rice size amount of toothpaste. for older children up to 6 years old use a pea size amount.

4. Parents should begin flossing their child's teeth as soon as their teeth start touching.

www.ingramcontent.com/pod-product-compliance
Lightning Source LLC
Chambersburg PA
CBHW040251220526
45473CB00001B/443